# KINGDOMKEY
# HEALTHCARE AGENCY'S
## COMPANY HANDBOOK

# TABLE OF CONTENTS


**Section One**
*Code of Conduct Protocol* . . . . . . . . . . . . . . . . . . . . . . . . 5

**Section Two**
*Documentation Policy* . . . . . . . . . . . . . . . . . . . . . . . . . . 9

**Section Three**
*Ohio HIPAA Law Policy* . . . . . . . . . . . . . . . . . . . . . . . . 13

**Section Four**
*Safety and Emergency Procedures* . . . . . . . . . . . . . . . . . . . 17

**Section Five**
*Dress Code Policy* . . . . . . . . . . . . . . . . . . . . . . . . . . . . 21

**Section Six**
*Timekeeping and Attendance* . . . . . . . . . . . . . . . . . . . . . 25

**Section Seven**
*Benefits and Leave Policies* . . . . . . . . . . . . . . . . . . . . . . . 29

**Section Eight**
*Payroll* . . . . . . . . . . . . . . . . . . . . . . . . . . . . . . . . . . . 33

**Section Nine**
*Training and Performance Policy* . . . . . . . . . . . . . . . . . . . 37

**Section Ten**

*Employee Conduct and Discipline Policy.* . . . . . . . . . . . . . . **41**

**Section Eleven**

*Grievance and Complaint* . . . . . . . . . . . . . . . . . . . . . . **45**

**Section Twelve**

*Termination and Resignation Policy*. . . . . . . . . . . . . . . . . . **49**

# CODE OF CONDUCT PROTOCOL

## 1. Professionalism:

- All staff members are expected to maintain a high level of professionalism in their interactions with clients, colleagues, and other individuals involved in the care process.
- Treat all individuals with respect, dignity, and empathy, regardless of their background or circumstances.

## 2. Confidentiality:

- Respect and maintain the confidentiality of client information, including personal, medical, and financial details.
- Only share client information with authorized individuals or organizations as required by law or with the client's explicit consent.

### 3. Ethical Behavior:

- Adhere to ethical standards and guidelines set forth by relevant professional bodies and regulatory authorities.
- Avoid conflicts of interest and ensure that personal relationships or interests do not compromise the quality of care provided.

### 4. Respect for Boundaries:

- Maintain appropriate professional boundaries with clients and their families.
- Avoid engaging in personal relationships or activities that may compromise the professional relationship or create conflicts of interest.

### 5. Safety and Well-being:

- Prioritize the safety and well-being of clients at all times.
- Follow established safety protocols and guidelines to prevent accidents, injuries, or any harm to clients.

### 6. Communication:

- Maintain clear and effective communication with clients, their families, and other healthcare professionals involved in the care process.
- Listen actively, respond promptly, and provide accurate and relevant information.

## 7. Continuous Professional Development:

- Commit to ongoing learning and professional development to enhance knowledge and skills.
- Stay updated on the latest industry trends, best practices, and regulatory requirements.

## 8. Reporting Concerns:

- Report any concerns, suspicions, or incidents of abuse, neglect, or unethical behavior to the appropriate authorities within the organization.
- Follow the established reporting protocols and ensure that all necessary documentation is provided.

## 9. Compliance with Policies and Procedures:

- Familiarize yourself with and adhere to all policies, procedures, and guidelines set forth by KingdomKey Healthcare Agency.
- Seek clarification or guidance if any policies or procedures are unclear or if you require further information.

## 10. Accountability:

- Take responsibility for your actions and decisions.
- Accept feedback, learn from mistakes, and strive for continuous improvement.

# DOCUMENTATION POLICY

## 1. Purpose:

- The purpose of this policy is to establish guidelines for the accurate and timely documentation of client care and related activities by staff members of KingdomKey Healthcare Agency's home care services.
- This policy ensures that documentation is comprehensive, consistent, and meets legal, regulatory, and organizational requirements.

## 2. Documentation Standards:

- All client care and related activities must be documented in a clear, accurate, and objective manner.
- Use only approved forms or electronic systems provided by KingdomKey Healthcare Agency for documentation purposes.

- Include relevant information such as date, time, location, client identification, and staff member's name or identification.

## 3. Timeliness:

- Documentation should be completed in a timely manner, preferably immediately after providing care or as soon as possible thereafter.
- Late entries should be clearly marked as such and include the reason for the delay.

## 4. Objective and Factual Information:

- Document observations, assessments, interventions, and outcomes in an objective and factual manner.
- Avoid subjective interpretations or assumptions.
- Use specific and descriptive language, avoiding vague or ambiguous terms.

## 5. Confidentiality and Privacy:

- Maintain the confidentiality and privacy of client information during the documentation process.
- Store and handle documentation in a secure manner to prevent unauthorized access or disclosure.

## 6. Signature and Authentication:

- All entries must be signed or electronically authenticated by the staff member responsible for the documentation.
- Signatures or electronic authentication should be legible, include the staff member's name and title, and indicate the date and time of the entry.

## 7. Corrections and Amendments:

- If an error is made in documentation, do not erase or delete the original entry.
- Cross out the incorrect information with a single line, write "error" or "correction," and provide the correct information.
- Include the date, time, and staff member's signature or authentication for the correction.

## 8. Communication and Collaboration:

- Document any communication or collaboration with other healthcare professionals, clients, or their families regarding the care provided.
- Include relevant information shared, decisions made, and any follow-up actions required.

## 9. Review and Auditing:

- Regularly review and audit documentation to ensure compliance with this policy and identify areas for improvement.
- Documented care should align with the agency's policies, procedures, and best practices.

## 10. Retention and Disposal:

- Follow the agency's retention and disposal policies for client care documentation.
- Retain documentation for the required period as per legal, regulatory, and organizational requirements.

# OHIO HIPAA LAW POLICY

## 1. Purpose:

- The purpose of this policy is to ensure compliance with the Health Insurance Portability and Accountability Act (HIPAA) and the Ohio state laws regarding the privacy and security of protected health information (PHI).
- This policy applies to all staff members, contractors, and volunteers of KingdomKey Healthcare Agency who handle or have access to PHI.

## 2. Definitions:

- Protected Health Information (PHI): Any individually identifiable health information, including demographic data, that is created, received, maintained, or transmitted by the agency.
- Covered Entity: KingdomKey Healthcare Agency is considered a covered entity under HIPAA.

- Business Associate: Any individual or organization that performs services on behalf of KingdomKey Healthcare Agency that involves the use or disclosure of PHI.

## 3. Privacy and Confidentiality:

- All staff members must respect and maintain the privacy and confidentiality of PHI.
- PHI should only be accessed or disclosed on a need-to-know basis for the purpose of providing care or as required by law.
- Staff members should not discuss or disclose PHI in public areas where unauthorized individuals may overhear.

## 4. Security Safeguards:

- KingdomKey Healthcare Agency will implement reasonable administrative, physical, and technical safeguards to protect PHI from unauthorized access, use, or disclosure.
- Staff members should follow established security protocols, such as password protection, encryption, and secure transmission methods, to safeguard PHI.

## 5. Use and Disclosure of PHI:

- PHI may only be used or disclosed for treatment, payment, and healthcare operations purposes, as permitted by HIPAA.

- Written authorization from the client is required for any other use or disclosure of PHI, unless otherwise permitted by law.

## 6. Minimum Necessary Standard:

- Staff members should only access, use, or disclose the minimum amount of PHI necessary to perform their job responsibilities.
- When sharing PHI with other healthcare providers or entities, staff members should ensure that only the necessary information is shared for the intended purpose.

## 7. Breach Notification:

- Any suspected or confirmed breach of unsecured PHI must be reported immediately to the designated Privacy Officer.
- The Privacy Officer will conduct a thorough investigation and follow the appropriate breach notification procedures as required by law.

## 8. Training and Awareness:

- All staff members will receive initial and ongoing training on HIPAA regulations, this policy, and related procedures.
- Staff members should stay updated on changes in HIPAA regulations and attend refresher training as required.

## 9. Business Associates:

- KingdomKey Healthcare Agency will enter into written agreements with business associates who handle PHI on behalf of the agency.
- Business associates must comply with HIPAA regulations and provide reasonable assurances of safeguarding PHI.

## 10. Policy Violations:

- Violations of this policy may result in disciplinary action, up to and including termination of employment or contract.
- Any suspected violations should be reported to the designated Privacy Officer.

# SAFETY AND EMERGENCY PROCEDURES

## 1. Purpose:

- The purpose of this policy is to establish safety and emergency procedures to ensure the well-being of staff members and clients during home care services provided by KingdomKey Healthcare Agency.
- This policy aims to prevent accidents, injuries, and minimize risks associated with emergencies.

## 2. Risk Assessment:

- Prior to providing care, staff members should conduct a risk assessment of the client's home environment to identify potential hazards or safety concerns.
- Document any identified risks and take appropriate measures to mitigate them.

## 3. Personal Safety:

- Staff members should prioritize their personal safety at all times.
- If a situation poses an immediate threat to personal safety, remove oneself from the situation and call for assistance as necessary.
- Staff members should not engage in any activities that exceed their training or comfort level.

## 4. Infection Control:

- Follow established infection control protocols, including hand hygiene, proper use of personal protective equipment (PPE), and disposal of contaminated materials.
- Educate clients and their families on infection prevention measures as appropriate.

## 5. Client Safety:

- Ensure the safety of clients during care provision by following best practices and utilizing appropriate assistive devices.
- Assess the client's mobility, fall risk, and environment to implement necessary precautions.
- Encourage clients to report any safety concerns or incidents promptly.

## 6. Fire Safety:

- Familiarize oneself with the location and operation of fire extinguishers, fire alarms, and emergency exits in the client's home.
- In the event of a fire, follow established evacuation procedures, assist clients as needed, and contact emergency services.

## 7. Medical Emergencies:

- In the event of a medical emergency, assess the situation, provide immediate assistance within the scope of training, and call emergency services.
- Document the details of the emergency, actions taken, and any communication with healthcare professionals or emergency responders.

## 8. Natural Disasters:

- Develop a plan for natural disasters, such as hurricanes, earthquakes, or severe weather events, in consultation with the client and their family.
- Ensure access to emergency supplies, such as food, water, medications, and a communication plan.

## 9. Reporting and Documentation:

- Promptly report any safety concerns, incidents, or near misses to the appropriate supervisor or management.
- Document safety-related incidents, actions taken, and any follow-up required.

## 10. Training and Education:

- Staff members should receive training on safety and emergency procedures during orientation and periodically thereafter.
- Stay updated on best practices, emergency response protocols, and any changes in safety regulations.

# DRESS CODE POLICY

## 1. Purpose:

- The purpose of this policy is to establish a dress code that promotes a professional and unified appearance for staff members of KingdomKey Healthcare Agency's home care services.
- This policy ensures that staff members present themselves in a manner that instills confidence and trust in the agency's services.

## 2. Acceptable Attire:

- Staff members are required to wear scrub sets in black, white, or red colors.
- KingdomKey Healthcare Agency branded attire, such as shirts or jackets, may also be worn as part of the uniform.
- Scrubs should be clean, well-fitted, and in good condition.

### 3. Footwear:

- Closed-toe shoes with non-slip soles must be worn for safety reasons.
- Shoes should be clean, comfortable, and appropriate for the tasks performed.

### 4. Personal Hygiene and Grooming:

- Staff members should maintain good personal hygiene and grooming practices.
- Hair should be clean, neatly groomed, and secured away from the face.
- Nails should be clean, trimmed, and free from excessive length or decorative elements.
- Avoid wearing excessive jewelry or accessories that may interfere with providing care.

### 5. Personal Protective Equipment (PPE):

- In addition to the dress code, staff members must adhere to any specific PPE requirements based on the nature of the care provided.
- This may include gloves, masks, gowns, or other protective items as necessary.

### 6. Exceptions and Special Circumstances:

- In certain situations, staff members may be allowed to deviate from the dress code for medical or religious reasons.
- Any requests for exceptions must be discussed with and approved by the appropriate supervisor or management.

## 7. Policy Compliance:

- All staff members are expected to comply with the dress code policy.
- Failure to adhere to the policy may result in corrective action, up to and including disciplinary measures.

## 8. Updates and Modifications:

- KingdomKey Healthcare Agency reserves the right to modify or update the dress code policy as necessary.
- Staff members will be notified of any changes and provided with sufficient time to comply.

# TIMEKEEPING AND ATTENDANCE

## 1. Purpose:

- The purpose of this policy is to establish guidelines for accurate timekeeping and attendance for Care Specialists of KingdomKey Healthcare Agency's home care services.
- This policy ensures that accurate records are maintained for proper payment and to monitor staff attendance.

## 2. Timekeeping System:

- All Care Specialists are required to use the CareCenta link for timekeeping purposes.
- Care Specialists must enable the GPS service on their cellphones, tablets, or iPad devices upon arrival at the client's home and after the completion of each shift.

## 3. Arrival and Departure:

- Care Specialists must log in to the CareCenta system upon arrival at the client's home and log out after completing the shift.
- This information will be used to verify attendance and calculate accurate payment.

## 4. Visit Notes and Documentation:

- Care Specialists are responsible for entering visit notes in the CareCenta system for each client visit.
- Visit notes should be detailed, accurate, and reflect the care provided during the visit.
- Care Specialists must complete the Care Specialist Visit Form, including any required documentation, and submit it for proper payment.

## 5. Compliance with Shift Schedule:

- Care Specialists are expected to adhere to their assigned shift schedules.
- Notify the appropriate supervisor or management in advance of any anticipated tardiness, absence, or change in schedule.

## 6. Punctuality and Attendance:

- Care Specialists are expected to arrive at the client's home on time and ready to provide care.
- Excessive tardiness or absenteeism may result in disciplinary action, up to and including termination of employment.

## 7. Overtime and Additional Hours:

- Care Specialists must obtain prior approval from the appropriate supervisor or management for any overtime or additional hours worked beyond their scheduled shifts.
- Unauthorized overtime may not be reimbursed.

## 8. Timekeeping Accuracy:

- Care Specialists are responsible for accurately recording their time worked in the CareCenta system.
- Any discrepancies or errors should be promptly reported to the appropriate supervisor or management for correction.

## 9. Confidentiality and Data Security:

- Care Specialists must ensure the confidentiality and security of any client information accessed through the CareCenta system.
- Do not share login credentials or access the system on unauthorized devices.

## 10. Policy Compliance:

- All Care Specialists are expected to comply with this Timekeeping and Attendance policy.
- Failure to adhere to the policy may result in corrective action, up to and including disciplinary measures.

# BENEFITS AND LEAVE POLICIES

## 1. Purpose:

- The purpose of this policy is to outline the benefits and leave policies provided to employees of KingdomKey Healthcare Agency's home care services.
- This policy ensures that employees are aware of the benefits they are entitled to and the procedures for requesting and utilizing leave.

## 2. Eligibility:

- All regular full-time employees are eligible for benefits and leave as outlined in this policy.
- Part-time employees may be eligible for certain benefits on a prorated basis, as determined by their employment status and applicable laws.

## 3. Health Insurance:

- KingdomKey Healthcare Agency provides eligible employees with access to a comprehensive health insurance plan.
- Employees may be required to contribute a portion of the premium based on their employment status and plan selection.

## 4. Paid Time Off (PTO):

- Employees accrue PTO based on their length of service and employment status.
- PTO can be used for vacation, personal time, or illness, as approved by the supervisor.
- The procedure for requesting and scheduling PTO should be followed, and requests should be submitted in advance whenever possible.

## 5. Sick Leave:

- Employees are entitled to sick leave for their own illness or medical appointments, or to care for an immediate family member.
- The amount of sick leave provided and the procedure for requesting and documenting sick leave should be followed.

## 6. Family and Medical Leave Act (FMLA):

- Eligible employees may be entitled to job-protected leave under the FMLA for qualifying reasons, such as the birth or adoption of a child, caring for a family member with a serious health condition, or the employee's own serious health condition.

- The procedure for requesting and documenting FMLA leave should be followed.

## 7. Bereavement Leave:

- Employees may be granted a certain number of days of paid bereavement leave in the event of the death of an immediate family member.
- The procedure for requesting and documenting bereavement leave should be followed.

## 8. Holidays:

- KingdomKey Healthcare Agency observes certain holidays and provides eligible employees with paid time off on those days.
- The specific holidays and eligibility criteria will be communicated to employees.

## 9. Retirement Plan:

- KingdomKey Healthcare Agency offers a retirement plan, such as a 401(k), to eligible employees.
- Employees may be eligible to contribute a portion of their salary to the plan, and the agency may provide a matching contribution.

## 10. Policy Updates:

- This Benefits and Leave Policies are not applicable for contractors and may be revised or updated from time to time.
- Employees will be notified of any changes and provided with updated policy information.

# PAYROLL

## 1. Purpose:

- The purpose of this policy is to establish guidelines for payroll processing and payment for employees of KingdomKey Healthcare Agency's home care services.
- This policy ensures timely and accurate payment to employees for their services rendered.

## 2. Payroll Schedule:

- Payroll will be processed on a weekly basis
- All client visit forms must be submitted by employees to the designated department by Friday of each week to receive payment for the following week.
-   - Payroll checks will be deposited on Thursdays.

## 3. Direct Deposit:

- KingdomKey Healthcare Agency utilizes direct deposit as the primary method of payment.

- All employees are required to provide their bank account information to the Payroll department for direct deposit setup.
- Payroll checks will be automatically deposited into employees' designated bank accounts on a weekly basis.

## 4. Payroll Deductions:

- Payroll deductions may be made in accordance with applicable laws, regulations, and employee agreements.
- Deductions may include but are not limited to taxes, healthcare benefits, retirement contributions, and any other authorized deductions.

## 5. Payroll Errors or Discrepancies:

- Employees should promptly report any payroll errors or discrepancies to the Payroll department.
- The Payroll department will investigate and rectify any errors or discrepancies as soon as possible.

## 6. Payroll Records:

- Accurate records of payroll information, including earnings, deductions, and tax withholdings, will be maintained by the Payroll department.

## 7. Payroll Confidentiality:

- Payroll information is considered confidential and will be handled with the utmost confidentiality and security.

- Access to payroll information will be restricted to authorized personnel for payroll processing and related purposes.

## 8. Policy Updates:

- This Payroll Policy may be revised or updated from time to time.
- Employees | Contractors will be notified of any changes and provided with updated policy information.

# TRAINING AND PERFORMANCE POLICY

## POLICY STATEMENT:

At KingdomKey Healthcare Agency, we are committed to providing high-quality home care services to our clients. We recognize that the training and development of our employees are crucial to maintaining the highest standards of care. This policy outlines our approach to training and performance management to ensure that our employees are well-equipped and continuously supported in delivering exceptional care.

## 1. Training and Development:

1.1. New Employee Orientation: All new employees will undergo a comprehensive orientation program that covers our agency's mission, values, policies, and procedures. This orientation will also include an introduction to the specific job responsibilities and expectations.

1.2. Job-Specific Training: Employees will receive job-specific training to ensure they possess the necessary skills and knowledge to perform their roles effectively. This training may include topics such as client care techniques, infection control, medication administration, and documentation.

1.3. Ongoing Training: We are committed to providing ongoing training opportunities to enhance the skills and knowledge of our employees. Regular training sessions, workshops, seminars, and online courses will be offered to address emerging trends, best practices, and regulatory updates in the home care industry.

1.4. Personal Development: We encourage our employees to pursue personal and professional growth. We will support their participation in relevant conferences, certifications, and educational programs that contribute to their career advancement and the improvement of our services.

## 2. Performance Management:

2.1. Performance Expectations: Clear performance expectations will be communicated to all employees. These expectations will align with our agency's values, quality standards, and regulatory requirements.

2.2. Performance Evaluation: Regular performance evaluations will be conducted to assess employee performance and identify areas for improvement. Evaluations will be based on objective criteria, such as client feedback, adherence to policies and procedures, and job-specific competencies.

2.3. Performance Feedback and Coaching: Supervisors will provide timely and constructive feedback to employees on their performance. This feedback will be used to recognize and reinforce positive performance and address areas needing improvement. Coaching and mentoring will be provided to support employees in achieving their performance goals.

2.4. Performance Improvement Plans: In cases where an employee's performance falls below expectations, a performance improvement plan may be implemented. This plan will outline specific goals, timelines, and support mechanisms to help the employee improve their performance. Regular follow-ups will be conducted to monitor progress.

## 3. Documentation and Record-Keeping:

3.1. Training Records: Accurate and up-to-date training records will be maintained for each employee. These records will include details of completed training programs, certifications, and ongoing professional development activities.

3.2.  Performance Evaluation Records: Performance evaluations and related documentation will be securely maintained as part of the employee's personnel file. These records will be treated with confidentiality and used for performance management purposes only.

## 4. Compliance:

4.1.  Regulatory Compliance: All training and performance management activities will comply with applicable federal, state, and local laws, regulations, and industry standards.

4.2.  Confidentiality and Privacy: Confidentiality and privacy will be maintained throughout the training and performance management process. Employee performance information will only be shared with authorized individuals on a need-to-know basis.

## 5. Review and Updates:

This Training and Performance Policy will be reviewed periodically to ensure its effectiveness and relevance. Updates will be made as necessary to reflect changes in industry standards, regulations, or agency requirements.

By implementing this Training and Performance Policy, KingdomKey Healthcare Agency aims to foster a culture of continuous learning, professional growth, and exceptional care among our employees.

# EMPLOYEE CONDUCT AND DISCIPLINE POLICY

## 1. Purpose:

- The purpose of this policy is to establish guidelines for employee conduct and discipline within KingdomKey Healthcare Agency's home care services.
- This policy outlines the expectations for employee behavior, the consequences of policy violations, and the disciplinary procedures to address misconduct.

## 2. Professional Conduct:

- Employees are expected to conduct themselves in a professional manner at all times while representing KingdomKey Healthcare Agency.
- This includes treating clients, their families, and colleagues with respect, maintaining confidentiality, and adhering to ethical standards.

## 3. Compliance with Policies and Regulations:

- Employees are required to comply with all applicable laws, regulations, and KingdomKey Healthcare Agency's policies and procedures.
- Failure to comply may result in disciplinary action, up to and including termination of employment.

## 4. Attendance and Punctuality:

- Employees are expected to report to work on time and maintain regular attendance.
- Excessive tardiness or absenteeism may result in disciplinary action, including verbal or written warnings, suspension, or termination.

## 5. Substance Abuse:

- The use, possession, or distribution of illegal drugs or alcohol while on duty is strictly prohibited.
- Employees found to be under the influence of drugs or alcohol may be subject to disciplinary action, up to and including termination.

## 6. Confidentiality and Privacy:

- Employees must maintain the confidentiality and privacy of client information, in accordance with applicable laws and regulations.
- Unauthorized disclosure or misuse of confidential information may result in disciplinary action.

## 7. Harassment and Discrimination:

- KingdomKey Healthcare Agency is committed to providing a work environment free from harassment and discrimination.
- Employees must not engage in any form of harassment or discrimination based on protected characteristics, such as race, gender, religion, or disability.
- Violations of this policy will be subject to disciplinary action, including investigation and appropriate corrective measures.

## 8. Use of Technology and Social Media:

- Employees should use technology, including company-provided devices and social media platforms, in a responsible and professional manner.
- Inappropriate use, such as accessing or sharing explicit content or engaging in cyberbullying, may result in disciplinary action.

## 9. Disciplinary Procedure:

- Any alleged misconduct will be investigated promptly and impartially.
- The disciplinary procedure may include verbal or written warnings, suspension, and termination, depending on the severity and recurrence of the violation.

## 10. Policy Acknowledgment:

- All employees are required to read and acknowledge receipt of this Employee Conduct and Discipline policy.
- By signing the acknowledgment, employees confirm their understanding of the policy and their commitment to comply with its provisions.

# GRIEVANCE AND COMPLAINT

## 1. Purpose:

- The purpose of this policy is to establish a fair and transparent process for addressing employee grievances and client complaints within KingdomKey Healthcare Agency's home care services.
- This policy aims to provide a mechanism for resolving concerns and improving the quality of care and working environment.

## 2. Grievance Procedure for Employees:

a. Informal Resolution:
   - Employees are encouraged to attempt an informal resolution by discussing the concern with their immediate supervisor or manager.
   - Supervisors should make every effort to address the grievance promptly and resolve it to the satisfaction of both parties.

b. Formal Grievance:
   - If the grievance is not resolved informally, the employee may submit a formal written grievance to the Human Resources department.
   - The written grievance should include a clear description of the issue, relevant facts, and any supporting documentation.
   - Human Resources will conduct a thorough investigation and provide a written response within a reasonable timeframe.

c. Appeal Process:
   - If the employee is not satisfied with the resolution provided by Human Resources, they may appeal the decision to the appropriate management level.
   - The appeal should be submitted in writing, outlining the reasons for the appeal and any additional information or evidence.
   - Management will review the appeal and provide a final decision, which will be communicated to the employee in writing.

## 3. Complaint Procedure for Clients:

a. Informal Resolution:
   - Clients or their representatives are encouraged to first discuss any concerns or complaints with the assigned Care Specialist or their immediate supervisor.
   - Every effort should be made to address the complaint promptly and resolve it to the satisfaction of the client.

b. Formal Complaint:
- If the complaint is not resolved informally, the client or their representative may submit a formal written complaint to the Client Services department.
- The written complaint should include a clear description of the issue, relevant facts, and any supporting documentation.
- Client Services will conduct a thorough investigation and provide a written response within a reasonable timeframe.

c. Appeal Process:
- If the client or their representative is not satisfied with the resolution provided by Client Services, they may appeal the decision to the appropriate management level.
- The appeal should be submitted in writing, outlining the reasons for the appeal and any additional information or evidence.
- Management will review the appeal and provide a final decision, which will be communicated to the client or their representative in writing.

## 4. Confidentiality:

- All grievances and complaints will be handled with the utmost confidentiality, to the extent permitted by law and organizational policies.
- Information related to the grievance or complaint will only be shared with individuals directly involved in the resolution process.

## 5. Non-Retaliation:

- KingdomKey Healthcare Agency prohibits retaliation against employees or clients who file grievances or complaints in good faith.
- Any form of retaliation will be subject to disciplinary action.

## 6. Policy Review:

- This Grievance and Complaint Procedures policy will be reviewed periodically to ensure its effectiveness and compliance with applicable laws and regulations.

# TERMINATION AND RESIGNATION POLICY

## 1. Purpose:

- The purpose of this policy is to establish guidelines for the termination of employment and resignation process within KingdomKey Healthcare Agency's home care services.
- This policy outlines the procedures to be followed by both the employee and the organization to ensure a smooth transition and protect the rights of all parties involved.

## 2. Termination of Employment:

a. Grounds for Termination:
- Employment with KingdomKey Healthcare Agency may be terminated for various reasons, including but not limited to:
  ◦ Violation of company policies or procedures

- Poor performance or failure to meet job expectations
- Misconduct or unethical behavior
- Insubordination or refusal to follow instructions
- Absenteeism or excessive tardiness
- Breach of confidentiality or privacy
- Any other behavior or action deemed detrimental to the organization or its clients

b. Termination Process:
- The termination process will be conducted in accordance with applicable laws and regulations.
- Human Resources will coordinate the termination process, ensuring that all necessary documentation and procedures are followed.
- The employee will be provided with a termination notice, which may include the reason for termination and the effective date of termination.
- Final wages and any applicable benefits or entitlements will be calculated and paid in accordance with applicable laws and company policies.

## 3. Resignation:

a. Notice Period:
- Employees are expected to provide a written notice of resignation to their immediate supervisor or manager.
- The notice period should be in accordance with the employment contract or applicable laws, but generally, a minimum of two weeks' notice is customary.

- In some cases, a longer notice period may be required, especially for key positions or to ensure a smooth transition of responsibilities.

b. Exit Interview:
  - Upon resignation, employees may be required to participate in an exit interview conducted by Human Resources.
  - The purpose of the exit interview is to gather feedback, address any concerns, and obtain information that may help improve the organization.

c. Return of Company Property:
  - Prior to the employee's departure, all company property, including but not limited to keys, identification badges, equipment, and confidential documents, must be returned to the organization.

## 4. Non-Compete and Confidentiality Agreements:

- Employees who have signed non-compete or confidentiality agreements are expected to comply with the terms of those agreements, even after termination or resignation.

## 5. Policy Violations:

- In the event of a policy violation during the notice period or resignation process, the organization reserves the right to take appropriate disciplinary action, which may include immediate termination.

## 6. References:

- KingdomKey Healthcare Agency will provide references for former employees upon request, in accordance with applicable laws and company policies.
- References will be provided based on accurate and objective information regarding the employee's job performance and conduct during their employment.

## 7. Policy Review:

- This Termination and Resignation Policy will be reviewed periodically to ensure its effectiveness and compliance with applicable laws and regulations.